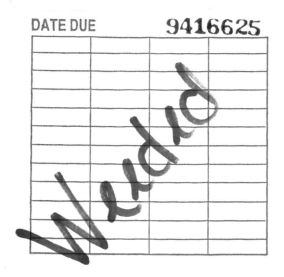

DATE DUE   9416625

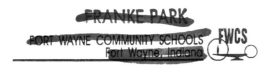

DEMCO

Be the Best
FUN &
FITNESS

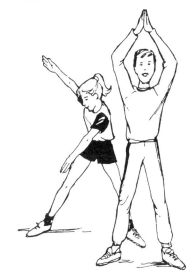

A Step-By-Step Guide
By Sheila Rich

9416625

Troll Associates

Library of Congress Cataloging-in-Publication Data

Rich, Sheila.
    Fun & fitness: a step-by-step guide / by Sheila Rich.
        p.   cm.—(Be the best!)
    Summary: Advice for starting and continuing a sound fitness
program.
    ISBN 0-8167-1949-7 (lib. bdg.)   ISBN 0-8167-1950-0 (pbk.)
    1. Physical fitness—Juvenile literature.   2. Exercise—Juvenile
literature.   [1. Physical fitness.   2. Exercise.]   I. Title.
II. Title: Fun and fitness.   III. Series.
GV481.R513   1990
613.7—dc20   89-27393

Be the Best

FUN & FITNESS

A Step-By-Step Guide

FOREWORD

by John Lemperle

Everyone wants to feel good. And well-rounded physical fitness exercises and activities are among the best ways to keep feeling good. Through them, you can develop strength and endurance. You can also enjoy greater freedom of movement and flexibility. Even how you see yourself, your self-image, will improve.

Follow the instructions in this book closely. If you do and you keep at it, you'll be well on your way to a lifetime of fun and fitness.

John R. Lemperle

John Lemperle has been an adaptive physical education officer for the United States Military Academy in West Point, New York, since 1967. For 13 years, he coached Army's triathlon (run, shoot, swim) team. John has also taught personal conditioning, swimming, racquetball, and squash. He has a master's degree in physical education from Idaho State University and has written half a dozen manuals for various fitness programs. From 1976 through 1978, and then again in 1980, John Lemperle won the masters division of the National Triathlon Championship.

Contents

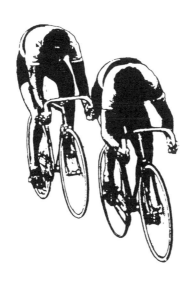

1

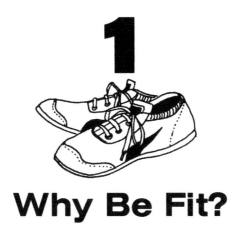

Why Be Fit?

Which is more fun: sitting around watching others play your favorite game, or actually playing the game yourself? Most people would agree that playing the game is more fun.

Physical fitness is a big part of any game or sport. If you are physically fit, you will be able to play longer without tiring. That will make you a better player and athlete. It will also make you feel better about the way you look and the way your body performs in almost everything you do.

Getting in shape and staying physically fit can help you live a longer and healthier life. This book will show you many ways to start and continue a sound fitness program. Being fit is fun. So join the crowd and get in shape!

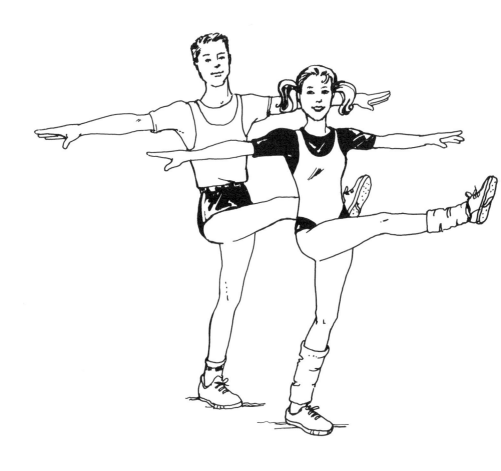

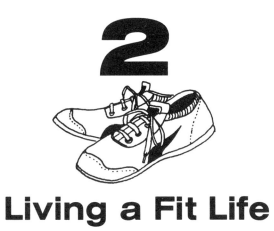

Living a Fit Life

Following a physical fitness program takes dedication. Sometimes it seems like hard work. But it can also be fun and give you a feeling of personal satisfaction. Remember, what you are building every time you work out is a better body. That body is yours and no one else's for life. Do right by it, and it'll do right by you.

Correct physical fitness is finding a program you enjoy so you'll do it on a regular basis. Some people like aerobics. Others like jogging. Some fitness buffs enjoy calisthenics. There is also rope jumping, isometrics, and fitness games. You can even do combinations of all of the above. The wide variety of activities is what makes getting in shape so much fun.

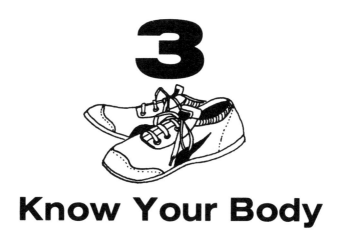

Know Your Body

Overall fitness is not just working out. It is also understanding a little about your body and how it works.

HOW MUSCLES WORK

Muscles are the machines that move your body. Like machines, muscles need fuel. Eating and breathing give muscles the fuel and air they need to work. Some fuel for muscle work is stored in the muscle itself. That fuel has a special name. It is called glycogen (gli-co-gin). Glycogen is also made and stored in the liver.

When glycogen is used up, your muscles start to tire. The better the physical condition you are in, the more glycogen you can store. Glycogen is the first source of muscle energy.

A second source of muscle energy is the fat and blood sugar delivered by the blood. Muscles use these when they're out of glycogen. You can restore glycogen or re-energize your muscles by eating right.

FOOD

A balanced diet is the best way to provide plenty of stored energy for your muscles. This means eating some combination of meat, fish, poultry, vegetables, and fruit. It also means eating breads and whole-grain cereals (oatmeal, bran, wheat) as well as drinking water and milk.

EAT A BALANCED DIET

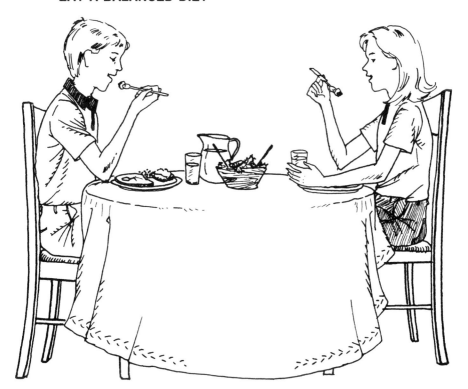

Junk foods aren't called that for nothing. They have low nutritional value, can lead to weight problems, and should generally be avoided. However, a candy bar or cookie can temporarily help your muscles during a hard workout. But much better snacks than those are fresh fruits (apples, pears, oranges, peaches) and even cold vegetables (carrots, celery, cucumbers).

OXYGEN

Oxygen is in the air we breathe. We use it to burn fuel. Carbon dioxide is a gas given off as muscles burn the fuel. The blood carries oxygen to the muscles as they work and then carries away carbon dioxide.

During activities like working out, your muscles need oxygen faster and give off carbon dioxide more quickly. That is why your breathing increases as you exercise.

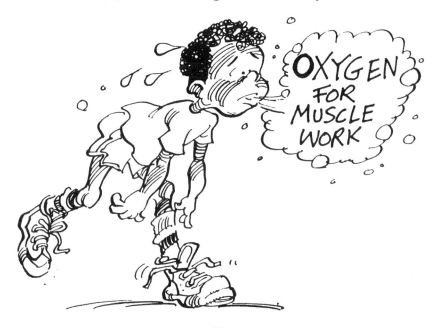

REST AND SLEEP

Some people think they must work out until they feel exhausted in order to benefit from exercise. They are wrong. Listen to your body. You will know when you are really tired. Once you are, let your body rest and recover. There is nothing wrong with taking a day off from your exercise program.

Getting enough sleep is another important way to restore energy and let your body recover from working out. An athlete should try to get eight to ten hours of sleep a night.

ENJOY 8 TO 10 HOURS OF SLEEP

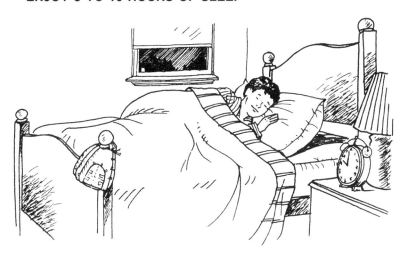

THE HEART

The heart is a very important muscle. It pumps blood through the body. Without it, other muscles can't receive fuel and oxygen or get rid of carbon dioxide and other waste products. Like any muscle, the heart can be strengthened by exercise. Endurance exercises like jogging, skipping rope, aerobics, and walking are good ways to strengthen the heart.

CALORIES AND LOSING WEIGHT

A calorie is the measure of energy produced by food. Calories are needed for fuel and used up during work-outs. Everyone burns or uses calories at a different rate. That is why some people can eat a lot and stay thin, while others eat the same amount and gain weight.

It takes 3,500 calories to make one pound of body weight. If you take in 7,000 calories and only burn up 3,500 calories, you will gain a pound. That is the real secret to losing or gaining weight.

The food you eat has calories. The exercise you do burns up a number of calories. If you use up 3,500 more calories than you take in, you will lose a pound. If you use up the same number of calories you take in, your weight will stay the same.

When you are working out, don't be afraid to drink water. It will help replace fluids lost while sweating, and it won't increase your weight.

4

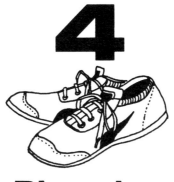

Planning
Your Workout

No serious exercise or fitness program should ever be started without first having a physical examination. Exercise is good for the heart. But it also makes the heart work hard. Make sure your heart is in good shape before you start to work out. A doctor can also help you plan a sensible program.

How many times a week you work out basically depends on you. Some people work out every day and feel good about it. Others work out every other day. Only you can decide what is best for you. A good rule of thumb is to do your workout at least three times a week.

Each workout can last from fifteen to sixty or more minutes, with periods of rest included. A good workout period is usually thirty to forty-five minutes long. This includes taking short, two- or three-minute rest periods when you feel tired.

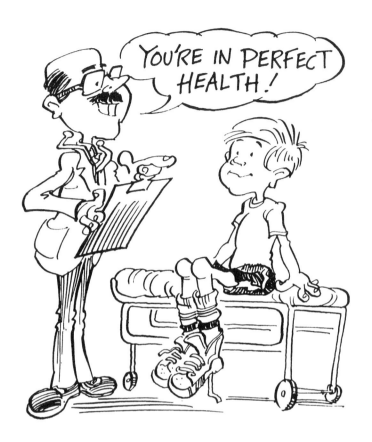

CLOTHES TO WORK OUT IN

Summer workout attire should be loose-fitting clothes. Shorts and a T-shirt are fine. So are sweat socks and sneakers.

For winter workouts, sweat pants, a sweat shirt, sweat socks, and sneakers are all you need. For outdoor work, you can also wear a Windbreaker and a wool cap.

Girls usually wear body suits or dance tights for aerobic work. You can also wear sneakers and sweat socks. Body suits are also fine for girls who do isometric or weight training.

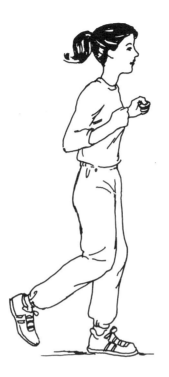

COMBINING PROGRAMS

To be totally fit, you need to combine exercises that build muscles with those that increase endurance. Calisthenics can be combined with jogging. Weightlifting can be done with rope skipping. Choose your exercises according to what you want to do with your body. You can also decide to improve a part of your body (for example, arms or legs), and focus on that.

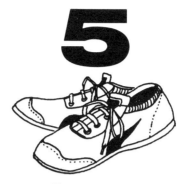

Basic Calisthenics

Calisthenics are light muscle-building exercises. They help tone your body and increase your strength. To a lesser degree, they also increase your endurance. And calisthenics can be done almost anywhere.

Every exercise you complete is called a repetition. The number of repetitions you do before resting or stopping is called a set. For each exercise, try to do two or three sets. How many repetitions you do in each set is up to you. Do not tire yourself out in the first set. Try to do between three and ten repetitions in each set. Make sure it is a comfortable number for you.

TUMMY TOUGHENERS

These exercises concentrate on hardening your stomach muscles. They will also make your waist trimmer.

Basic Sit-Up To start, lie on your back on the floor. Keep your knees bent at a ninety-degree angle and keep your arms at your sides. Curl your head and raise your torso forty-five degrees toward your chest. Return to the starting position. As you get stronger, increase the repetitions in each set.

To make the basic sit-up harder, place your hands behind your neck. Keep them there throughout the exercise. You can also trim your waist by touching an elbow to the opposite knee when you sit up. Alternate side to side.

SIT-UPS

BASIC SIT-UP

A. Arms at side, legs bent at knees with feet flat on floor

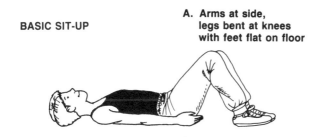

HARDER SIT-UP

B. Hands behind neck.

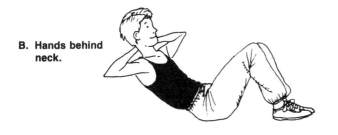

V Raise This version of a sit-up is guaranteed to make your stomach tough and hard. Again, start flat on your back. Stretch your arms out behind your head and keep your legs straight. Bring your upper and lower body off the ground at the same time so that you are balancing on your seat. Stretch forward, trying to touch your toes with your fingertips. Bring your body into a V position. Hold the V position for a count, then slowly drop back to the starting position. But stop if you feel pain.

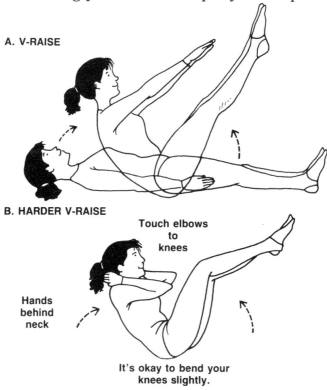

A. V-RAISE

B. HARDER V-RAISE

Touch elbows to knees

Hands behind neck

It's okay to bend your knees slightly.

Another version of this exercise is to lock your hands behind your neck and to try touching your elbows to your knees when you're in the V position. You can make the touch by bending your legs at the knees.

Leg Lifts   To begin, lie flat on your back. Keep your legs straight and together. Put your hands under your seat, with your palms on the floor. Raise your heels off the ground and hold them about ten inches off the floor. Try not to bend your knees. Hold your feet up for a count of eight to ten, then lower them. Discontinue if you feel back pain.

LEG LIFTS

A. BASIC

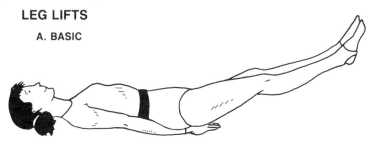

With hands under seat,
raise heels.
Hold position,
then lower.

B. HARD

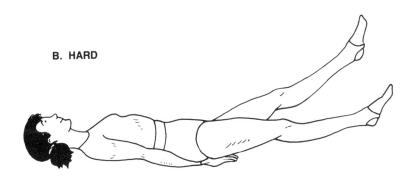

With hands under seat and
heels raised, open legs.
Hold position, then close legs.
Hold position, then lower.

A more difficult version of the leg-lift exercise is to raise your heels for a count of five. But this time, do not lower your feet to the floor. Spread your legs while they're in the air, and hold them open for a count of five. Then close your legs and hold them up for another count of five before lowering them.

Side Bending Stand with your feet spread about shoulder width. Lock your hands behind your neck, pointing your elbows out to the sides. Keeping your torso straight, bend sideways at the waist and move your left elbow toward your left hip. Hold for a count, then return to the starting position. Now bend to the right, lowering your right elbow toward your right hip. Hold and then return to the up position. That completes one repetition.

SIDE BENDING

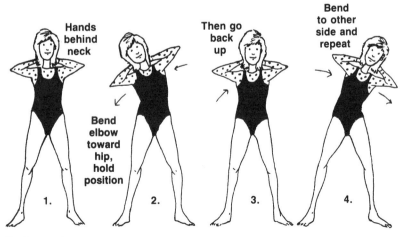

Hands behind neck

Bend elbow toward hip, hold position

Then go back up

Bend to other side and repeat

1.　2.　3.　4.

Feet spread

UPPER BODY BUILDERS

The following calisthenics will help strengthen the muscles in your arms and chest.

Basic Pushup Lie face down on the floor, keeping your legs together. Place your hands flat on the floor just under your shoulders, with your fingers spread and pointing forward. Place the balls of your feet and toes flat on the floor so your heels are pointing up.

Push your body off the floor by straightening your arms. As you rise, keep your back and legs straight and your chin up. Your weight should be on your hands and the balls of your feet. Your back remains straight.

Push up until your arms are all the way extended. Lower your body until your chest touches the floor. Then push up again. Continue in this fashion as many times as you can.

BASIC PUSHUP

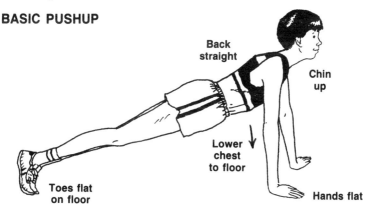

Back straight

Chin up

Lower chest to floor

Toes flat on floor

Hands flat

Knee Pushup The starting position for the knee pushup is almost exactly the same as the previously described pushup except for how you hold your legs.

KNEE PUSHUP

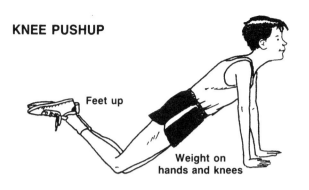

Feet up

Weight on hands and knees

Lie flat on your stomach with your hands under your shoulders. Keep your legs together, but bend them at the knees so your calves (the muscles in the lower part of your leg) and feet are up in the air behind you. As you extend your arms to push up, your weight is now on your hands *and* knees. Complete the knee pushup the same way as a basic pushup.

Chin-Ups Chin-ups require the use of an additional piece of equipment. An adjustable chinning bar that fits in doorways can be bought at most sporting goods stores. However, many parks, playgrounds, and school yards have chinning bars.

Grip the bar with your knuckles facing away from your body. Place your hands about shoulder width apart. You should be able to hang from the bar with your feet off the ground.

Pull your body up until your chin is above the bar. It's not easy to do! If you cannot get your chin above the bar, go up as far as you can.

Next, lower your body all the way down again. Do it slowly. Do not just drop down. Keep your body steady as you go up and down. Do not let it swing.

CHIN-UP

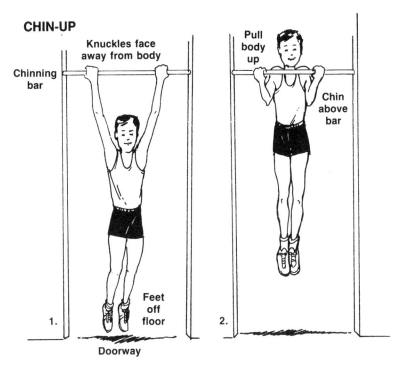

Chinning bar

Knuckles face away from body

Pull body up

Chin above bar

Feet off floor

1.

2.

Doorway

Modified Chin-Up Since a chinning bar is adjustable, you can lower it to do a modified chin-up. This is a bit easier than a regular chin-up.

MODIFIED CHIN-UP

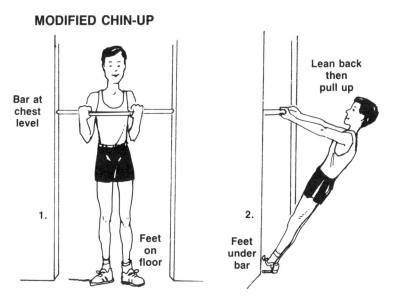

Bar at chest level

Lean back then pull up

Feet on floor

Feet under bar

1.

2.

Lower the bar to chest level. Stand and face the bar, grabbing it in regular chin-up fashion. Holding on tightly, lean back until your arms are extended. The heels of your feet will be on the floor under the bar. Your toes should rise off the floor and point up.

From that starting position, pull yourself up until your chest touches the bar. After you touch the bar, slowly lower yourself back to the starting position.

Arm Circles   Arm circles are a simple and easy exercise to do. Stand straight and tall. Extend your arms straight out to the sides, with the palms of your hands facing the ceiling.

While holding your arms out, rotate them in a circular motion backwards for a minute or so. Stop and then rotate the arms in a circular motion forward for a minute or so. Keep the circles you make small.

ARM CIRCLES

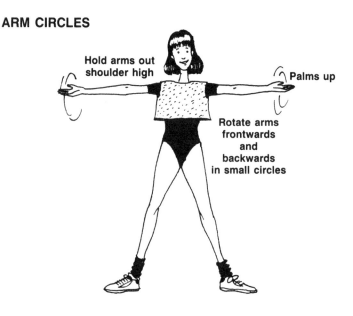

Hold arms out
shoulder high

Palms up

Rotate arms
frontwards
and
backwards
in small circles

Wing Stretchers   While standing straight, raise your forearms up in front of your torso. Keep your hands in front of your chest with your elbows pointed out. Your forearms and hands should form a straight line across your chest. Curl your hands into fists.

To do the wing stretcher, strongly thrust your elbows backwards three times in a row. Pause and then repeat. Remember to keep your arms up with your elbows at shoulder height.

WING STRETCHERS

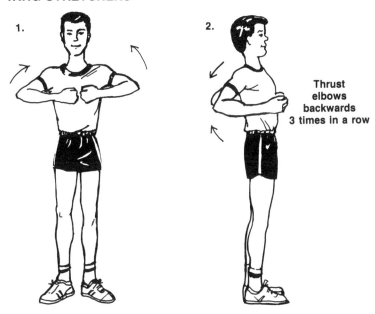

MORE BODY BUILDERS

The exercises that follow will develop several sets of muscles at the same time, including those in the back, legs, and shoulders. Many of these exercises will also benefit your chest, arms, and waist, as well as build endurance.

WINDMILL

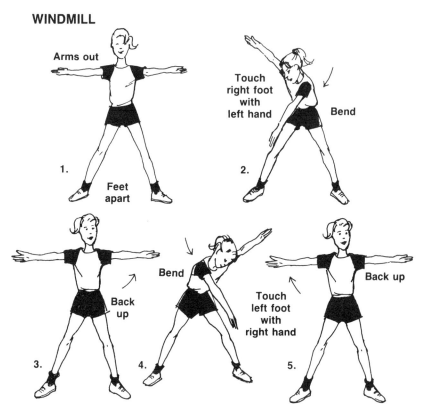

Arms out

1.

Feet apart

Touch right foot with left hand

Bend

2.

Back up

Back up

3.

Bend

Touch left foot with right hand

4.

Back up

5.

Windmills   The windmill exercise is sometimes called the alternate toe touch. It is an easy and fun exercise. To do the windmill, stand with your feet spread about shoulder width. Extend your arms straight out to the sides.

Bend and turn at the waist so your left hand reaches down and touches your right foot. Return to the straight-up position. Without pausing, bend and turn at the waist so your right hand reaches down and touches your left foot. Go back up again and continue.

As you touch your toes with your opposite hands and alternate side to side, your arms will look a little like a windmill. This is how the exercise got its name.

Jumping Jacks   To start a jumping jack, stand straight and tall with your arms at your sides and your legs together. That is the closed position.

Then do a little jump straight up. As you jump, spread your legs to about shoulder width. At the same time, raise your arms up at your sides and bend them slightly at the elbows so you can touch your fingertips together over your head. That is the open position.

Do another little skip jump, closing your legs and lowering your arms to your sides. Go back and forth in the closed and open positions as you bounce. Each time you return to the closed position, you will have completed one jumping jack. Do as many as you can before tiring or getting winded.

JUMPING JACKS

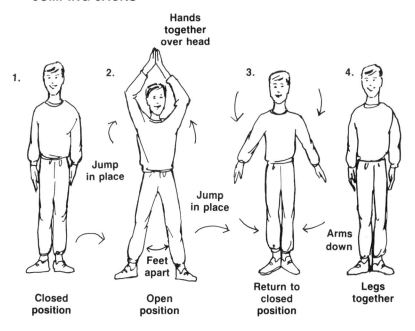

1. Closed position
2. Open position
3. Return to closed position
4. Legs together

Hands together over head

Jump in place

Feet apart

Jump in place

Arms down

Leg Elevators   Begin leg elevators by lying on your back. Put your arms at your sides and keep your legs together. Now bend your knees and draw your heels up to your seat, putting your feet flat on the floor.

Start the exercise by lifting your feet off the floor and raising your knees up toward your chest. Your arms should stay at your sides. When your feet are up with your knees at your chest, extend your legs so they point straight up. Hold them up for a count. Then bend your knees and lower your feet to the floor.

Back Arch   Lie face down on the floor. Point your toes and keep your legs together. Then put your hands behind your neck and interlock your fingers.

Slowly tense your lower back muscles so you lift your chest and your lower legs off the ground. Your body should rest on your stomach and thighs (the thick upper parts of your legs). Hold this arched position for a count, then return to a lying down position.

Boys may find it easier to do this exercise by putting their arms at their sides and tucking their hands (palms up) under their thighs. That way, their thighs will rest on their hands.

BACK ARCH

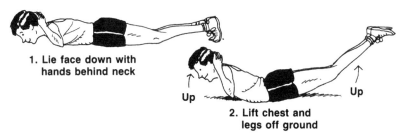

1. Lie face down with hands behind neck

Up

2. Lift chest and legs off ground

Up

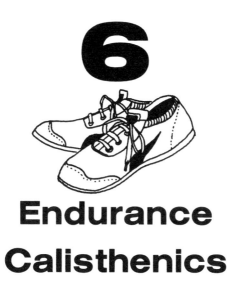

Endurance
Calisthenics

The calisthenics that follow will help you increase your endurance and also build the muscles in your legs.

RUNNING IN PLACE

There is nothing fancy about running in place. In a way, it's running without going anywhere. Instead of moving forward, you just stay in one place.

As you run in place, try to get your knees up very high. But do not go real fast at first. Run at a comfortable pace, pumping your arms. If you want, you can curl your hands into fists while running in place. Gradually go faster, then finish by slowing down again. Try to run in place for several minutes.

BICYCLE EXERCISE

The bicycle exercise uses the same pedaling movement you would use while riding a real bike. However, the bicycle exercise is done while lying on your back. This is another exercise in which you don't go anywhere.

Begin on your back. Raise your lower body off the floor by lifting your legs and hips off the ground. Keeping your elbows on the floor, put your hands on your hips. Use your elbows to help hold up your lower body.

With your legs in the air above your chest, start pedaling as if you were riding an imaginary bike. Bend one leg at the knee, lowering it to your chest, and then extend your leg so your foot shoots straight up. As one leg goes up, the other goes down. Do this exercise for several minutes.

BICYCLE EXERCISE

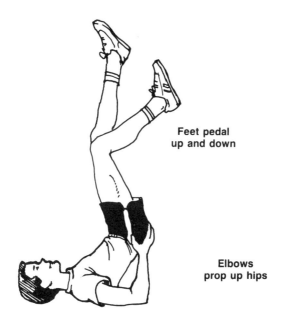

Feet pedal
up and down

Elbows
prop up hips

SPRINTER EXERCISE

To do the sprinter exercise, start in a pushup position (see page 23). Lie flat on your stomach, with your legs straight and your palms on the floor near your shoulders. Now straighten your arms so your body is in the "up" position.

While in this "up" position, bring your right knee up toward your chest so your foot is under your body. Your left leg should be extended with your foot way back behind you. By bouncing up slightly, reverse the position of your legs. As your hips bounce up, slide your left knee back into an extended position. Keep bouncing and reversing the position of your legs for several minutes.

SPRINTER EXERCISE

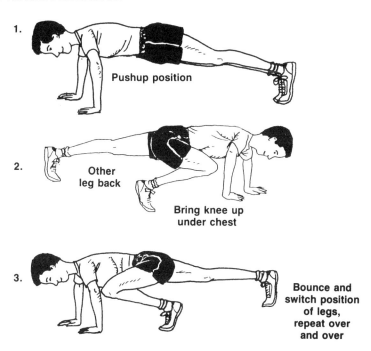

1. Pushup position

2. Other leg back / Bring knee up under chest

3. Bounce and switch position of legs, repeat over and over

33

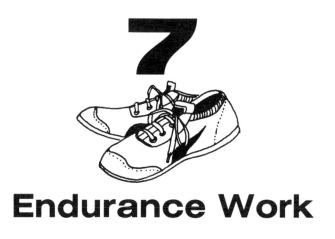

Endurance Work

Conditioning is very important to overall fitness. It benefits your entire body, especially your heart muscle. Here are some of the most popular exercises for conditioning.

WALKING

Believe it or not, simple walking is one of the best conditioning and heart exercises you can do. Walking a mile or more a day is very good exercise.

When walking for conditioning, remember to walk at a steady pace. Try to walk quickly, taking long, graceful strides. As you walk, swing your arms and breathe normally.

STRETCHING BEFORE JOGGING

Jogging or distance running at a slow, comfortable pace is an excellent way to increase stamina and build endurance. Before doing any kind of running, though, you should always prepare your muscles by stretching them first. Two stretches you can do are the crossed-leg stretch and the inner-thigh stretch.

Crossed-Leg Stretch To begin this stretch, stand straight with your hands at your sides. Cross your left leg over your right, placing your left foot beside the outside part of your right foot. *Slowly* bend forward at the waist and reach down with your hands to touch your toes. Stay in the down position for a count of three. Come back up and repeat several times. Uncross your legs, then cross the right leg over the left to reverse positions. Bend again. Remember, always do your stretching slowly.

CROSSED-LEG STRETCH

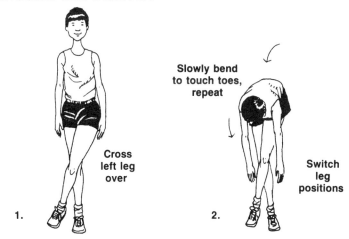

Slowly bend to touch toes, repeat

Cross left leg over

Switch leg positions

1.

2.

Inner-Thigh Stretch   To start this stretch, sit down. Bend your knees and place the soles of your feet together. Use your hands to help keep your heels close together. While sitting erect and keeping your feet together, lower your knees out to the sides. Get them as close to the floor as possible. Hold that position for a count of three before bringing the knees back up. Again, work slowly.

INNER-THIGH STRETCH

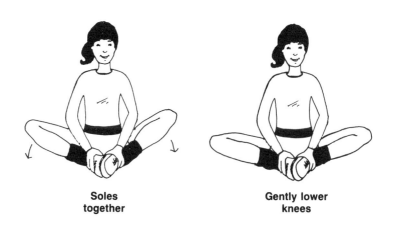

Soles
together

Gently lower
knees

JOGGING

Having limbered up by stretching, you are now ready to jog. When you jog, you are running for distance. You should not be concerned about speed or time.

An important difference between jogging and sprinting is the part of the runner's foot that touches the ground first after a stride. In jogging, the runner's heel touches the ground first, followed by the front of the foot.

36

The arm swing is also important. Run relaxed. Keep your hands open while jogging. Do not ball your hands into fists. Swing your arms in a comfortable manner. And do not swing your arms too far back or too high up in the front. Swinging your arms up about waist high and back to the hip is a good motion.

JOGGING

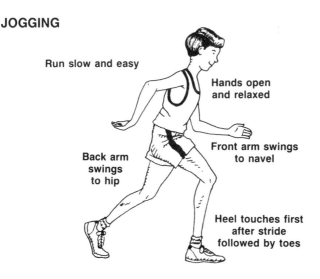

Run slow and easy

Hands open and relaxed

Back arm swings to hip

Front arm swings to navel

Heel touches first after stride followed by toes

Recommended places to jog are on tracks, around football or soccer fields, or in any open grassy area. Jogging on a sidewalk is okay. But there could be a problem with jogging on any hard surface that does not give slightly when your foot comes down. You may develop shin splints. These are aches and soreness in the sides of your lower legs. To avoid shin splints, try to jog on grass, dirt, or a track surface.

When you start jogging, set a realistic daily goal. Do not try to go too far. Jog until you are tired, then walk a little and rest. But always try to finish what you started out to do. Do not get tired and just stop jogging.

A good beginning distance to jog is a half mile. Gradually increase your distance to a full mile. After a while, try to jog between one mile and three miles. You do not have to jog the same distance every time.

Many people prefer to jog with a partner. Others prefer running at different places on different workout days. Both can make jogging more fun to do. But whatever way you like to jog, always try to jog at least three times a week.

SPRINTING

Sprinting is a good way to build your endurance while improving your foot speed and quickness. A sprint is a short, fast run. As with jogging, always start by first stretching your muscles.

When you sprint, the fronts, or balls, of your feet should hit the ground first after a stride. Your arm swing should also be higher in the front and more forceful than a jogger's swing.

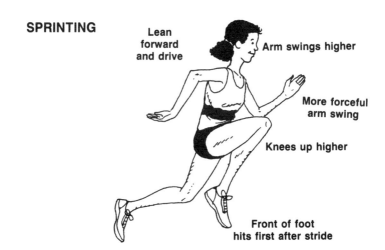

SPRINTING

Lean forward and drive

Arm swings higher

More forceful arm swing

Knees up higher

Front of foot hits first after stride

To sprint, start fast and get to top speed as quickly as possible. Run all the way past the finish line, then stop and jog or walk back to the starting line. Sprints should be done in sets like calisthenics. The walk or jog back gives you a chance to rest and recover. Try to do sets of three to five sprints each workout.

A good distance for workout sprints is thirty-five to forty yards. You can also sprint increased distances of fifty to sixty yards if you like. But never sprint on hard surfaces like a sidewalk or pavement. That is a sure way to get shin splints.

JUMPING ROPE

For this exercise, the first thing you'll need is a jump rope. Jump ropes usually have swiveling wooden handles and are available at most sporting goods stores for a reasonable price. You can also use an old length of clothesline rope. Shorten it to a comfortable length by wrapping it around your hands.

In jumping rope, you can work by jumping sets or jumping for a certain period. When doing sets, try to jump between thirty and a hundred times in each set. If you miss, pause a second and begin again. Start with the number where you missed. After each set, rest. Then move on to the next set.

When jumping rope for time, set a goal of, say, three minutes. That means you will be spending three minutes jumping rope, not including rest time. Jump rope for one minute and quickly start again if you miss. When the minute is up, rest until you feel recovered. Start again and jump for another minute. Then rest and do another minute. If these one-minute intervals are too hard for you at first, try jumping rope in half-minute intervals.

When jumping rope by yourself, you can use either a two-foot jump or an alternating foot jump.

JUMPING ROPE

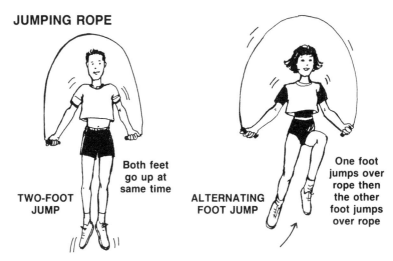

Two-Foot Jump   This isn't too difficult. However, once you start to feel tired, it gets harder and harder. Stand straight, spreading your feet slightly or keeping them together if you like. As the rope passes under you, jump with both feet at the same time. But don't jump too high. Try to jump as long as you can without missing.

Alternating Foot Jump   The alternating foot jump is like running in place (see page 31) while jumping rope. Only one foot jumps over the rope at a time. Your feet should alternate skipping over the rope (right, left, right, etc.) as you run in place. To make the alternating foot jump harder, raise your knees high as you skip.

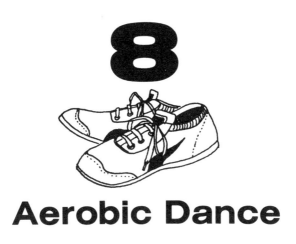

Aerobic Dance

The word *aerobic* means "living or occurring only in the presence of oxygen." An aerobic exercise is an exercise done long enough to get your muscles to use a greater amount of oxygen than they normally do. Many of the exercises already described qualify as aerobic exercises. They help you to breathe better. This allows your heart (see page 13) to do less work, which is good.

Aerobic dance can help improve your coordination, stamina, rhythm, and agility. The exercise movements making up aerobic dance are done one after another to music. Normally, an aerobic dance lasts from two to five minutes for beginners. Advanced aerobic dancers work longer. Either way, the main idea of aerobics is to keep moving!

Different types of aerobic dance movements will be described here. To form a dance routine, you must string together several of these movements. But before you do, learn each movement without music. And remember that aerobic dance is fun for both girls and boys.

WARM-UP STRETCHES

Before starting to dance, you should always loosen up by stretching. The crossed-leg stretch (see page 35) and the inner-thigh stretch (see page 36) are good ways to loosen up. Another effective warm-up stretch is the ankle-hold stretch.

Begin the ankle-hold stretch by standing with your feet apart. Raise your right leg and bend it at the knee so that your heel is lifted toward your left hip. Grab your right ankle with your left hand and hold your leg up.

ANKLE-HOLD STRETCH

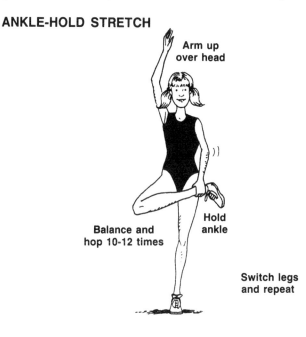

Arm up
over head

Hold
ankle

Balance and
hop 10-12 times

Switch legs
and repeat

Raise your right hand straight up over your head. While balancing on one foot, hop up and down ten to twelve times. Put your foot down and do the same with the other leg. Repeat with both legs several times.

LUNGE MOVE

Start the lunge move by standing straight. Next, turn toward your left. Lunge by stepping in that direction with your left foot, keeping the leg slightly bent at the knee. Leave the right leg extended behind you. Lift your right heel so that the toes of your right foot are pointed toward the floor.

At the same time, extend your right hand out with the palm up. Your left hand should go on your left hip. Turn right and stop. Stand straight and then lunge right. Now step with the right foot. Leave the left foot behind you, keeping your left leg extended. Point the toe. Then reach out with your left hand, keeping your right hand on your right hip.

LUNGES

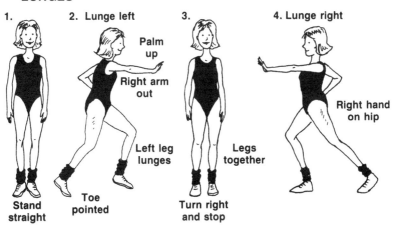

1. Stand straight

2. Lunge left
Palm up
Right arm out
Left leg lunges
Toe pointed

3. Legs together
Turn right and stop

4. Lunge right
Right hand on hip

STEP SLIDERS

To begin a step slide to the right, stand straight and put your left hand on your left hip. Extend your right arm straight out at the side about shoulder high. Point your fingers up.

Now slide your right foot out away from your body about shoulder width, and point the toe. Transfer your weight to the right foot. Then let your left foot glide over to your right so the heels of your feet come together while the toes remain slightly apart. Once your feet are together, clap your hands.

Next, put your right hand on your right hip. Extend your left hand out to the side. Slide your left foot away from your body. Transfer your weight to the left foot. Glide your right foot over to join your left foot at the heels. Keep your toes slightly apart. Again, clap your hands.

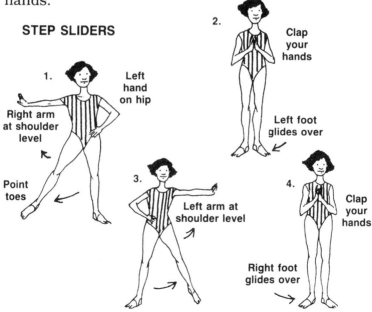

STEP SLIDERS

1. Left hand on hip
   Right arm at shoulder level
   Point toes

2. Clap your hands
   Left foot glides over

3. Left arm at shoulder level

4. Clap your hands
   Right foot glides over

CROSS KICK

The cross kick isn't really hard to do. But you must keep your balance while doing it.

Begin by standing with your arms straight out to the sides at shoulder level. Move forward by taking a step with your right foot. As you do, lift your left leg. Keep the left leg straight with the toe pointed, then swing it up across your right leg in a kicking motion. Your kick should go about waist high.

Bring your left leg down. Take another step with the right foot and cross kick with the left again. Bring the leg down. This time, step with the left and cross kick with the right leg. Do the same kick again. Repeat these cross kicks in sets of two.

CROSS KICK

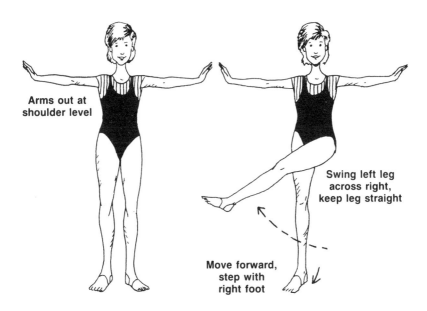

Arms out at shoulder level

Swing left leg across right, keep leg straight

Move forward, step with right foot

CANCAN KICK

Begin by standing with your feet spread shoulder width and your toes pointed out to the sides just slightly. Hold your arms straight out to the sides. Lift your right knee straight up to about waist high, then put your foot back on the floor.

Next, bring your hands down to touch your palms together in front of your lower belly. As you do, swing your right leg across your left knee, kicking out to the left side. Then bring your right leg back down to the start position.

Now put your arms back out to the sides at shoulder level. Bring your left knee straight up to about waist high, then put it down. Lower your arms to touch your palms in front of your stomach again. Swing your left leg across the right knee and kick out to the right side.

Return to the starting position. Keeping your arms out to the sides, lift your right knee up on the right side under the elbow. When your knee is about waist high, kick out sideways to your right. As you do, lower your arms and touch your palms together in front of your waist.

Again, return to the starting position. Now do the same movement to the left. With your arms out to the sides, raise your left knee out to the left side under the left elbow. Kick out to the left side. As you do, lower your arms and touch your palms in front of your waist.

That completes the cancan kick. It may seem hard to do. But once you learn it, it's really fun!

CANCAN KICK

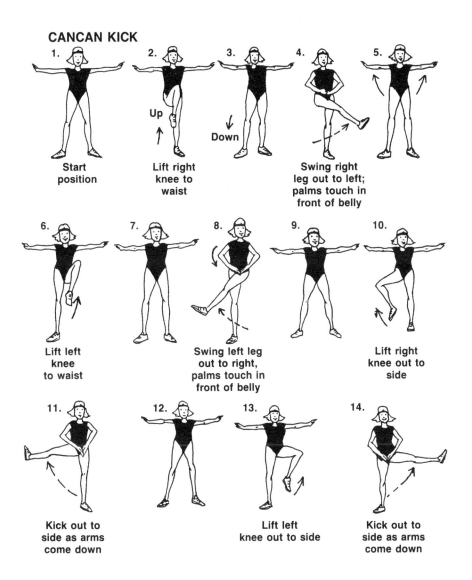

1. Start position

2. Lift right knee to waist

3. Up / Down

4. Swing right leg out to left; palms touch in front of belly

5.

6. Lift left knee to waist

7.

8. Swing left leg out to right, palms touch in front of belly

9.

10. Lift right knee out to side

11. Kick out to side as arms come down

12.

13. Lift left knee out to side

14. Kick out to side as arms come down

SIDE CLAPS

To begin a side clap, stand straight with your feet together. Extend your arms straight out sideways at shoulder level. Turn your head to look to the right. Drop your right shoulder so that your right arm tilts down and your left arm tilts up.

47

Take a short step to the right, keeping your right toe pointed. After a very brief pause, close your feet by moving your left foot toward the right. Bring your heels together, but keep your toes apart. When your feet come together, bring your hands down and clap them.

Now put your arms back out to the sides. Drop your left shoulder so that your left arm tilts down and your right arm tilts up. Step to the left, keeping the toe pointed. Pause and then close your heels together. Bring your hands down and clap them again.

SIDE CLAP

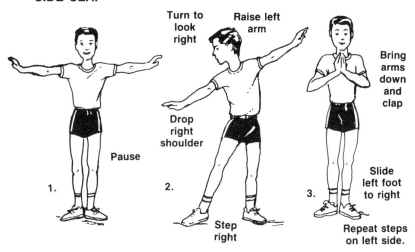

CROSS STEP

Begin the cross step by standing with your hands on your hips and your feet spread about shoulder width. Take a short step sideways to the right with your right foot. Now step sideways to the right with your left foot by crossing your left leg over in front of your right knee. Step to the right side with your right foot again. Then step to the right side with your left foot, this time crossing your left leg *behind* your right knee. Step to the right with your right foot in order to return to the starting position.

Now you'll take a cross step the other way. Take a short step sideways to the left with your left foot. Step to the left with your right leg crossing over in front of your left knee. Step to the left with your left foot. Then step to the left side with your right foot, crossing your right leg behind your left knee. Now do it all over one more time. That's how to do the cross step.

CROSS STEP TO RIGHT

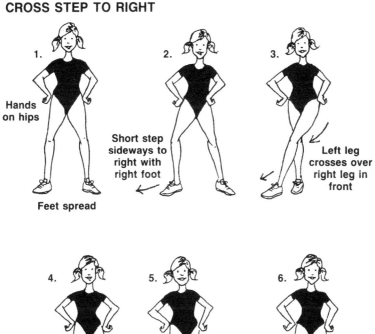

1. Hands on hips / Feet spread
2. Short step sideways to right with right foot
3. Left leg crosses over right leg in front

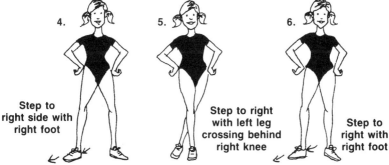

4. Step to right side with right foot
5. Step to right with left leg crossing behind right knee
6. Step to right with right foot

LEG TAPS

Once again, begin by standing with your feet spread shoulder width and with your arms held straight out to the sides at shoulder level. Kick your right leg out sideways to the left so that it crosses over your left leg. As your right leg swings up, lower your left hand and gently tap the calf part of your right leg with the palm of your left hand.

LEG TAPS

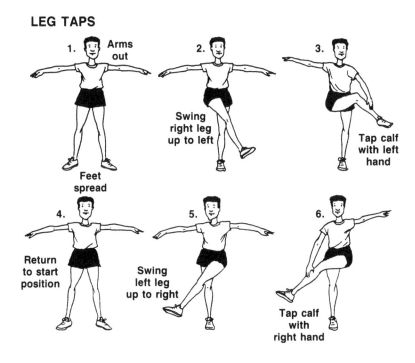

1. Arms out / Feet spread

2. Swing right leg up to left

3. Tap calf with left hand

4. Return to start position

5. Swing left leg up to right

6. Tap calf with right hand

Return to the start position. Now kick your left leg out sideways to the right so that it crosses over your right leg. Bring your right arm down as your left leg swings up, and tap the palm of your right hand against your left calf. Make sure you keep your other arm out and straight.

COOLING DOWN

What is a cool down? It is a period of light, easy exercises done after you finish a long period of hard exercises. Cooling down helps your body and muscles slow down gradually and relax.

For cooling down, you can use the crossed-leg stretch (see page 35), the inner-thigh stretch (see page 36), or the ankle-hold stretch (see page 42). You can also do these cooling down exercises:

Stand and Sway This is an easy way to cool down. Just spread your feet about shoulder width and raise your hands above your head. Then bend your arms slightly at the elbows so that your fingertips touch. Now lean your hips to the right as you slowly bend at the waist, lowering your upper body to the left. Without any pause, bring your upper body straight up and lean to the right as your hips shift left. Go back and forth several times.

Seated Windmill Sit down on the floor and spread your legs into a V position. Now stretch your arms out to the sides. Keeping your legs spread, reach over with your right hand to touch your left foot. Bring your right hand back, returning to the starting position. With your left hand, reach over to touch your right foot. Then bring back your left hand. Do these seated windmills several times slowly.

9

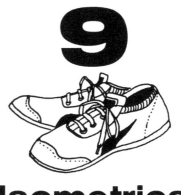

Isometrics

Isometric exercises take very little time and can be done anywhere. They help increase muscle strength but not endurance.

The purpose of isometrics is to exercise a muscle by pushing or pulling against an immovable object such as a wall. You can also do isometrics by having one muscle in your body work against another muscle.

One caution, though: Never keep the muscle you are exercising tensed for more than an eight-second count.

When starting isometrics, do not use your full strength. Use only about half of your strength for the first several weeks. Also, if you have any muscle pain at all while doing an isometric exercise, that means you are using too much force. Use less force immediately. If pain continues, stop and do not do that exercise anymore. If need be, have an adult help you with your isometric exercises.

ARM BUILDER

Stand with your feet apart and bend your right arm at the elbow, bringing your forearm up in front of you. Hold your forearm up about waist high and keep your right palm up.

Turn the palm of your left hand down and place it on top of your right hand. Lock your hands together. Now try to curl your right hand up toward your right shoulder. At the same time, use pressure from your left hand to hold your right hand down. Hold for a count of eight. Reverse the positions of your hands. Now use your right hand to hold your left hand down as your left arm tries to curl toward your left shoulder.

ISOMETRIC ARM BUILDER

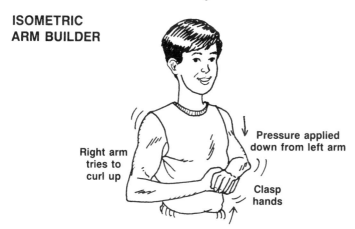

Pressure applied down from left arm

Right arm tries to curl up

Clasp hands

ARMS AND CHEST PUSH AND PULL

Stand with your feet apart. Raise your arms up in front of your chest, holding your elbows out to the sides. Place the palms of your hands together. Lock the fingers around your hands. Press your hands together forcefully and hold for eight seconds.

Keep your arms in the same position, but switch the position of your hands. Curl your fingers, using them to lock your hands together. Now pull out with your arms as if to separate your hands. Hold for a count of eight.

**ARMS AND CHEST
PUSH AND PULL**

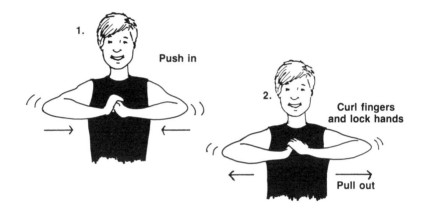

UPPER BODY BUILDER

Face a wall and stand about six inches from it. Place the palms of your hands flat against the wall just below your hips. Your fingers should point toward the floor. Press hard against the wall, keeping your arms straight, and hold.

Now turn so your back is to the wall. Place your palms against the wall the same way as before. Remember, point your fingertips down. Press backward against the wall as hard as you can, again keeping your arms straight.

For other ways to develop your upper body, see pages 23-27.

UPPER BODY BUILDER

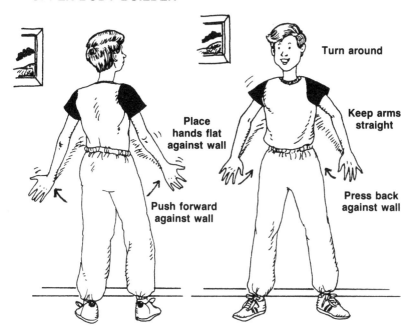

Turn around

Place hands flat against wall

Keep arms straight

Push forward against wall

Press back against wall

SIDE RAISE

To begin this exercise, stand in an open doorway so that your arms face the sides. Put your hands at your sides, with your palms facing your legs. Move your hands out so that the backs of your hands are against the door frame. Press out against the door frame as hard as you can. Try to hold for a count of eight.

TUMMY TENSER

Start in a standing position with your feet spread about shoulder width. Bend slightly at the waist and knees so that you can rest your hands on your knees (right hand on right knee, left hand on left knee). Keep your head and chin up. Concentrate and tense your stomach muscles. Try to make your stomach very hard. Take it easy and slowly at first. Do not try to make your stomach hurt. Hold for a few seconds, then relax.

See pages 18-22 for those calisthenics that will also toughen your tummy.

SIDE RAISE

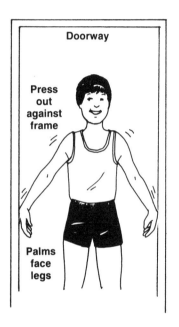

Doorway

Press out against frame

Palms face legs

TUMMY TENSER

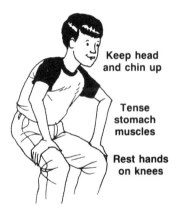

Keep head and chin up

Tense stomach muscles

Rest hands on knees

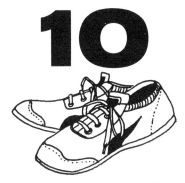

Fun Fitness Games

The following games and contests are ways to have extra fun while exercising and testing your strength, agility, and endurance.

ARM-WRESTLING MATCH

You and someone else sit at opposite ends of a table facing each other. Place your elbows on the table with your forearms and hands pointed up. Clasp hands so that both of your forearms are straight up. The object is to push your opponent's hand down so his or her knuckles touch the table top. You should push in the direction your palm is facing. As soon as the back of one person's hand touches the table, the match is over. Once the match starts, you cannot get up or move from your seat.

ARM-WRESTLING MATCH

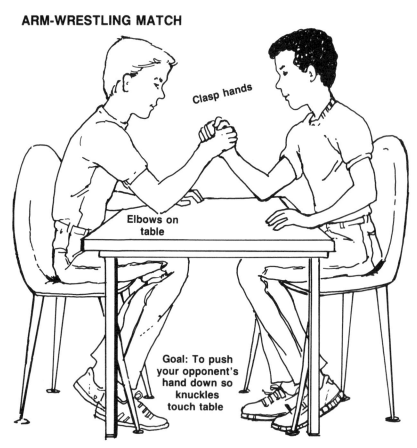

Clasp hands

Elbows on table

Goal: To push your opponent's hand down so knuckles touch table

PUSH OVER

This is another contest for two people. Stand straight and face your opponent so that the two of you are toe to toe. Your feet should be no more than shoulder width. Put your hands out just above your waist. Your palms should be facing your opponent and your fingers pointing up. Now press your palms against your opponent's palms.

The goal is to push your opponent off balance, *not* to knock him or her over onto the ground. The first one to move a step, no matter how small, is the loser.

58

PUSH OVER

Goal: to push your
opponent
off balance

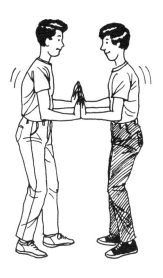

TOWEL TUG OF WAR

For this two-person contest, first tightly roll up an old towel. Next, draw a line in the dirt or on the sidewalk. You stand on one side of the line and your opponent stands on the other.

TOWEL TUG OF WAR

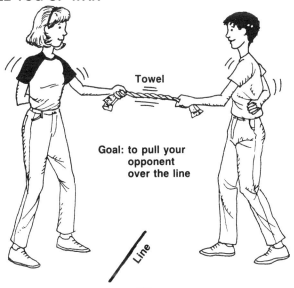

Towel

Goal: to pull your
opponent
over the line

Line

Grab onto an end of the towel with one hand and stretch it over the line so your opponent can grab the other end. Place your free hand behind your back. The object is to pull your opponent over the line. Anyone who steps over the line or lets go of the towel loses.

DUCK-WALK RACE

This is a race where two or more people can have a lot of fun. First, draw a start and a finish line. Stand at the starting line and put your hands on your hips. Squat down by bending your knees. To do the duck walk, swing your leg out to the side first and then forward.

The object of the duck-walk race is to stay in that squat position and cross the finish line first. Standing up is not allowed. And if you fall over, get up and start again! But stop if you feel pain.

DUCK-WALK RACE

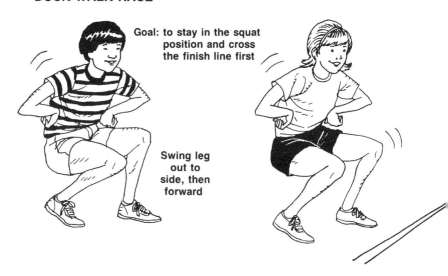

Goal: to stay in the squat position and cross the finish line first

Swing leg out to side, then forward

WHEELBARROW RACE

Four or more people in multiples of two can enjoy this race. It should be done only on the grass. This is a contest requiring strength and teamwork to win.

Begin by drawing a start and a finish line. One person gets in a pushup position (see page 23), with arms extended. That person is the wheelbarrow. The teammate of that person is the wheelbarrow pusher. He or she grabs the wheelbarrow's legs at the ankles and lifts up the wheelbarrow's feet. The wheelbarrow must balance up on his or her arms.

WHEELBARROW RACE

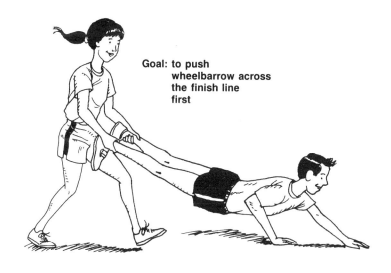

Goal: to push wheelbarrow across the finish line first

The object of this race is to push the wheelbarrow across the finish line first. The pusher must go slowly and carefully, allowing the wheelbarrow to walk and balance on his or her hands.

KANGAROO HOP

The kangaroo hop is a race two or more people can take part in. Again, draw a start and a finish line. At the starting line, fold your arms together across your chest. Squat down by bending your knees and lowering your seat toward your heels.

The object of this race is to stay in that position, bounce up and down like a kangaroo as fast as you can, and cross the finish line first.

KANGAROO HOP

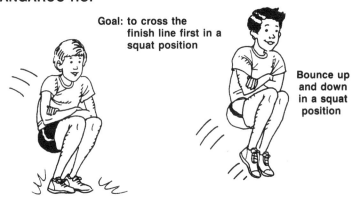

Goal: to cross the finish line first in a squat position

Bounce up and down in a squat position

11

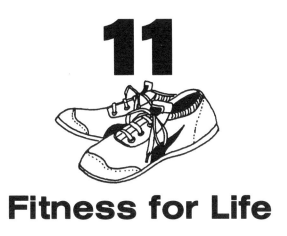

Fitness for Life

Doing instead of watching—that's what staying fit means. There are many ways you can stay fit that you may not even think of as exercise. A game of tag is exercise. So is skipping stones across a pond. Even climbing the stairs in your home is exercise.

Everyone needs exercise. How you exercise and how often you exercise are up to you. But keep as active as you can. It can help you live a healthier, longer, happier life. So be fit and have fun staying that way!

INDEX